Aerobics: A Guide to Keeping Your Heart and Body Healthy

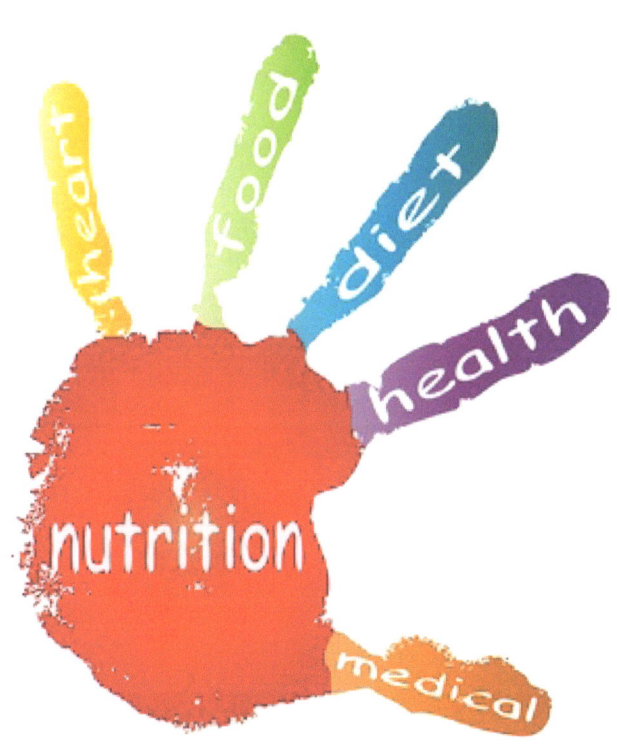

Cindy Wright

Aerobics: A Guide to Keeping Your Heart and Body Healthy

Cindy Wright
Copyright © 2013 by Cindy Wright.

This book was printed in the United Kingdom.

To order additional copies of this book, contact:

Email: cindys.great.books@gmail.com
Website: http://www.cindys-ebooks.webplusshop.com

Also by Cindy Wright

Travelling Through the Emerald Isle

The Popular Seaside Places of the United Kingdom

Worlds of Ice

Part of Your World

Addition Package

The Dark Traveller

Christmas Magic for Children

The Different Ways of Celebrating Easter

CONTENTS

What Is Aerobics?

Aerobics, which literally means "with oxygen", are exercises used to lose weight and regain health. There are many types of aerobic exercise, and if you do them daily, you will soon notice that you are healthier. Aerobics done at moderate levels of intensity for longer periods of time target the body parts you wish to slim. There are many advantages of aerobics, which is why this form of exercise is both important and popular among health-conscious people.

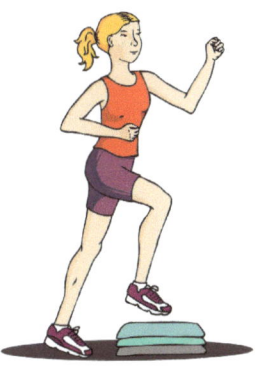

Exercise can be broken down into two categories: aerobic and anaerobic. These differ due to how the muscles contract during exercise, and how energy works within them.

Examples of anaerobic exercise include weight training or strength training. With aerobic exercises, even the well-built bodybuilder will not be able to run, swim, etc. for long periods.

During aerobics, you do not use bursts of energy. Instead, you spread out moderate levels of energy over longer periods to trigger the use of fat in energy production. In general, things such as long distance running, dancing and swimming are aerobic exercises, whereas sprinting, which uses short bursts of motion, is not.

The benefits of aerobic exercises are great, which is why most doctors recommend them to patients, even if they have a normal weight. Some of these benefits include strengthening the repertory muscles, enlarging the heart to pump more efficiently, improving oxygen and blood flow and increasing endurance.

Therefore, there is no reason for people not to do aerobics! There are a number of great exercise programs available, which include individual and class activities with groups. However, before you start any kind of new health care routine, it is important to learn how exactly aerobics works. You can do this in a number of ways.

• Primarily, you need to talk to your doctor if you want to make the best possible health decisions. A doctor will inform you about programs that are not beneficial for your body, that are too difficult or that could cause injury. He will also explain the best aerobic exercises, maybe recommend a personal trainer and stress the great health benefits of aerobics. The first stop should therefore be your doctor's surgery. Make sure you have enough time to ask all the questions you may have.

• The Internet is also a great resource when it comes to finding information on aerobics. You can read articles about its benefits, its history, interact in chat rooms and forums to share experiences and ask questions. The Internet can also let you look at specific routines and there are several websites that may help you put some routines together to suit your level and experience.

- Beyond the Internet, you can learn about aerobics using the traditional literature on the subject. Your local library should have a variety of books that you can read. If the resources there are out-dated, try the nearest bookshop. Always check online for discounted prices before purchasing a book you like.

- Fitness magazines are valuable, too. The information in there may not be published by professionals, but health care workers have checked the articles written in these magazines.

Learning about aerobics is not difficult. People are beginning to feel more health conscious, so that information is becoming more and more available.

Aerobics can decrease the risk of death due to cardiovascular problems, and can prevent the onset of osteoporosis in both men and women.

If you exercise regularly, you will be able to tolerate the challenges that life throws at you. For instance, it will help you fight against heart disease, reduce the risk of high blood pressure, osteoporosis, breast and colon cancer, depression, anxiety and stress. Aerobics are the key to a healthier and physically productive life, so do not wait another day before starting building a new and healthier you.

Exercise Is For Any Age Group

Everyone wants to get healthier, and everyone knows that when it comes down to it, doing aerobics on a regular basis can take you from being unhealthy to healthy, so you can enjoy all that life has to offer you. This goes for everyone, but there are certain groups of people who have to design their exercise very carefully to avoid injury.

Seniors are one of these groups of people. When it comes to aerobics for seniors, you must consider several things. Remember, aerobic exercise is something you must build on. You need to start small, depending on how healthy you are to begin with. If you want to get healthier, you have to start at the very bottom with basic work, and slowly build up on it. This is especially recommended for seniors. Take a health inventory before exercising on a daily basis. Seniors are prone to health problems, so they must see a doctor for a health check immediately.

However, after getting the all clear from a doctor, seniors can begin aerobic exercise the same as any person of any age. Think about what you want to achieve in aerobics, which will help you find your starting level. As long as it is not overdone, an aerobic workout will be beneficial to you.

REMEMBER: Discuss your plans with a doctor, even if you feel healthy. He will have more information about the types of exercise that will be the best for you.

Intensity and Endurance

Aerobics are great for losing weight and staying healthy, because they strengthen your breathing and heart and burn fat at the same time. Many people do not know or understand how to do an aerobics workout in order to maximize the results. Intensity is the key to any workout, so stick to these three rules in order to get the most out of it.

First, find the intensity that is comfortable for you. If you work out too intensely you may be injured or not get results. However, if you do not work out intensely enough, you will still not lose weight or become stronger. Therefore, you have to work with a program that has just the right intensity for you. When trying new exercises, try to make sure that they include enough weights or speed to make the workout hard, but not impossible. Remember that you will need to change the intensity of your workout as your tolerance and endurance increase. Check your routine about every one or two weeks to make sure it is still working for you.

The second rule to intensity is to be safe. Over-training is a huge problem, because it puts you and those around you in danger. When you under-train you will have no results, which may push you to intensify. That is good, but too much and you will be vomiting before it is over and possibly causing yourself injury. If you are training properly, your muscles should be sore, but your joints should not.

Never do an intense workout where you cannot control your form or breathing. Instead, take breaks and use lower weights or speed to get you back on track. This method will help you get more out of your workout. If injury occurs during a workout, call for help if people are near you. It is always a good idea to work with a partner or in a class.

Lastly, build intensity instead of jumping in the deep end. When you are starting to exercise, you will not be able to run the London Marathon! Building up slowly will help prevent injury, and lessen the frustration. Slowly building up your exercise routine will give you more success overall.

No matter what your current state of being in shape might be, it is always important to improve. You hear of aerobic workouts developed by people who have not worked out in years and are not in good shape. However, there are people who want to develop workouts who already do athletic work, like endurance athletes. They already know the basics of aerobics and simply want to get you in shape.

If you have been working out for a long time, or if you play a sport that requires you to have long periods of endurance, you probably know that aerobic workouts are also very important. In order for you be in the best shape possible, you have to be able to have your heart rate and breathing rate up accomplished by aerobics. However, if you are an athlete, chances are that the basic class is going to be boring for you, and is not going to benefit you at all. If you want to get in shape there are several things you can do.

First, the point of doing aerobics is to get your heart rate going and your breathing rate up. That means that if you are already an endurance athlete, you are going to have to find ways to push yourself past what you are able to do. If you are used to long distance running, and do not get winded, you are going to have to try and run faster or farther in order to get you heart rate going higher.

You have to be sure that you can find different ways to work out to challenge your body. You will have to increase the speed, or add something to your workout so that you can complete it in a way that challenges your body.

Remember that challenging your body is the point of doing aerobic workouts. Therefore, you have to find ways that your body is not used to working, and force it to work in that harder way.

Home, Classes or Gym

Beginners

If you are just getting started with aerobics, you might be feeling overwhelmed by all this information. It is true that there are many ways to work out, and if you can find a good program for you, you will become much healthier. You need to have a workout in which your body is moving fast, and your heart and lungs must be working hard to keep up. Do not think you have to start at the top straight away. You must work your way up to advanced aerobics. This can include running or marching in place with a series of movements that may seem intimidating to start with. Moreover, it is not safe to start anywhere other than as a beginner, because you may hurt yourself.

Beginner's aerobics are very easy and they are something you can do at home, especially if you are not ready for a group. The point is get your blood flowing. A great thing to do is starting by walking or jogging in place. You can move your arms up and down. The point of aerobics is to get your heart going, and the best way to do this is jumping jacks, for as many repetitions as you can do. This is the best way for you to start with aerobic training, because you are able to work up from nothing and really get in good shape. You can gradually proceed to doing more and more movements and faster.

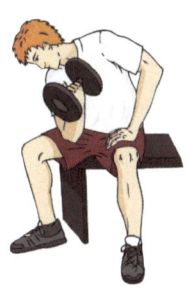

Something else you should keep in mind is that aerobics often works better to music. The way it works is to use the music to keep your tempo and keep you working hard. You can also time your exercises to music – like one set for an entire song, for instance. Music can be your motivator, and help you to keep working out.

Other examples to get you started, if you are able to do them, are brisk walking, cycling, swimming, yoga and Pilates.

Aerobics At Home

There are many ways you can make aerobics work for you. First, it is important that you understand how vital aerobic workouts are to your health. You can get healthy just by walking and by lifting weights (If you do not have weights compromise by using tins of carrots or something similar). In order to be truly healthy, you have to get your heart pumping and your blood flowing. This is why aerobic exercise is very important to you – it allows you to get all parts of the body working together.

However, sometimes you cannot go to the gym or take classes in order to get healthier. Many people are busy with family and job commitments, and going to these places does not fit their needs.

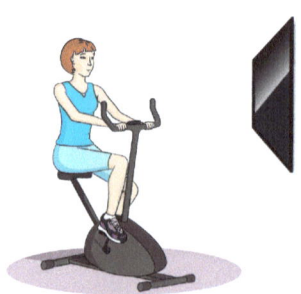

There are many things that you can do in order to work out at home. The fundamentals of aerobics, as we have already learned, are to get the heart pumping and breathing rate up.

The first and the most popular way to do it would be to get a bike or a treadmill in your house. You can put it in a convenient place and have it ready for when you have time to work out.

Another great thing is to develop a routine for yourself that includes running in place, skipping or even running around the block. All of these are important, because you can customize your workout to fit your needs.

When working out at home you must keep a record or a diary of your progress. This way you can monitor yourself, and make any changes necessary as you improve. Do not exercise within two hours of eating a meal or drink any alcohol or smoke cigarettes etc. before a workout. If you begin to feel short of breath or lightheaded, make sure you stop and rest for a while. If your condition does not improve, consult a doctor immediately.

Always make sure you start with a warm up. You can try some simple stretches of each muscle group. Your muscles must be warm to work properly and prevent injury. You can then move on to walking on the spot or light jogging to get your heart rate up. Once you have achieved this, you can move on to your planned workout. Remember to cool down with stretches, and deep slow breathing to bring your heart back to normal. Record your daily heart rates in your diary to notice the results.

Aerobic Classes

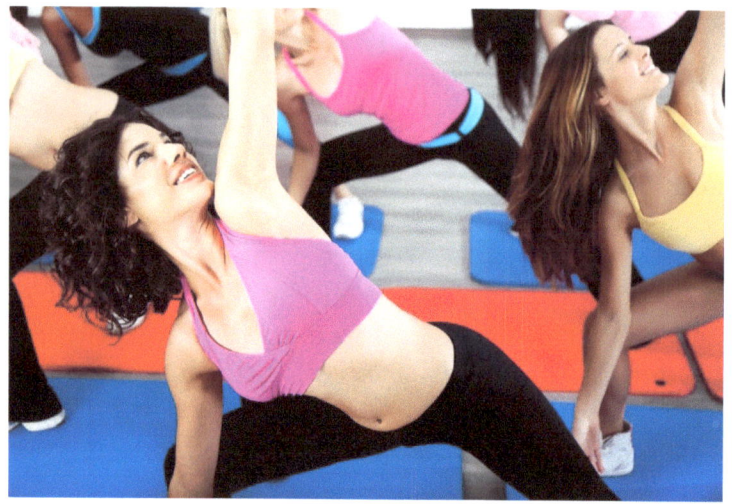

With aerobics, you will find that you can stay trimmer, have more endurance/stamina and participate in other physical activities for longer. One of the ways to do this is to join some classes, as you will be motivated to stick to it. You can also meet people who are at the same level as you, so hopefully you will not feel intimidated and have fun. Training of the fundamentals of working out is essential, as well as learning new moves so you can generally enjoy yourself. The class instructor should be experienced in their field, to help you gain the most out of your workout.

Everyone knows that the hardest part of exercising is motivating yourself into actually doing it, go to the gym or get your bike out. Signing up for an aerobics class schedules you to do this, and helps you not put it off. If you lack motivation, working out on your own may not be the answer. A class may be more beneficial for you.

Personal Trainers

There are many times in your life when you may need the help of a personal trainer, and doing aerobics is one of them. With the help of a trainer, you will reach your fitness goals quicker, and know how to maintain them. It is easy to find a trainer, but you need to find one you are comfortable with and who understands your needs. A trainer that stresses you out might sound good, but you could end up getting frustrated and not be at your best. Worst still, you could end up quitting aerobics altogether.

The point of having a personal trainer is so that you can be yourself, and be able to do your best when left alone. Your trainer can only help you with so much; you are the one who has to put the hard work in. He will encourage you, but allow you to work at your own pace.

A personal trainer will motivate you, and you will definitely get the work done. Therefore, there will be no putting it off until another time. If your trainer is willing to help you with any conditions you may have, you will be very happy with the results.

Aerobic Machines

When it comes to aerobics, you may find that you get better on a machine instead of walking, running or skipping. Aerobics have to adapt to your body and what is best for your health. Work closely with your doctor and trainer. They will help you make sure you do the best for your body and mind.

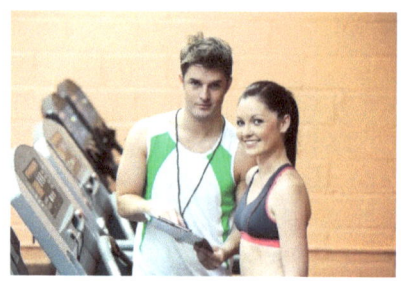

Machines have become very popular for working out on. They are easy to use and get used to. You do not have to worry about the cold, wet weather or finding the time to work out as you can fit one in your home. The easiest and most popular machines are a bike or a treadmill. You can work out on these no matter what time it is or what the weather is like. As long as you work out the same way, by getting your heart and breathing rate up slowly, this type of exercise could get you the results quicker. In addition, it is a lot more convenient than going to the gym. On the other hand, if you can get to a gym, there will be other people there, and maybe your very own personal trainer, as discussed in the last section, to help give you encouragement.

Choosing Suitable Clothing

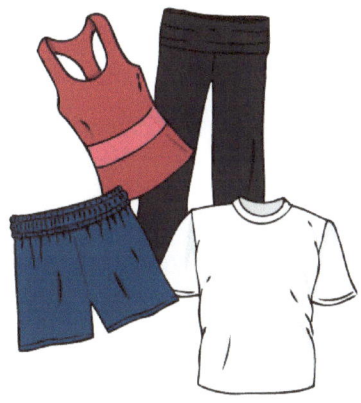

As mentioned in the sections above, aerobic exercise today is essential for healthy living. It can help you lose weight, and tone your muscles, giving them greater flexibility. The advantages are that this type of exercise works indoors and outdoors, at any time. It will also make you versatile in your skill and intensity level. It is even suitable for people who have never done any exercise in their life, who now want to take up a regular exercise program, as well as those of you who are dedicated sports fanatics.

To make all this happen, you must make sure you wear suitable clothing. They must be loose, but not ill fitting, avoid plastic and rubber, as these materials make your body temperature rise to harmful levels, wear many light layers instead of a heavy one, and wear light colours in the summer months, as these absorb heat slower.

If you are a beginner who is new to aerobics or any kind of exercise, it is very important to feel comfortable. Loose fitting clothes allow free airflow, whereas tight clothes restrict your movements, making the routine useless and possible causing injury. When buying your clothes, touch the material to see how it feels.   If the material is soft, you will have better flexibility.

If you like to be stylish, and fashion-conscious, make sure the material is comfortable. If you cannot move correctly, you will lose your motivation quickly. Do not spend too much either. Ask a gym instructor or a friend about how much your first outfit should cost.

The material that touches your skin should be able to absorb moisture. You could wear t-shirts, sweatshirts, joggers, tracksuit bottoms or tights.   If you wear proper clothing, your spirits and motivation get a boost, making your workout enjoyable.

FOCUS ON EFFORT, NOT DISCOMFORT!

Injuries

Aerobics are great exercises to lose weight, build endurance and stay heart healthy, but there is a downside. If you do not exercise carefully, you could injure yourself. So follow these few tips to make sure your workout stays fun and healthy.

First, consider your clothes. Good workout shoes are also important. Aerobics require a lot of movement. If your shoes are old, or the laces undo easily, you may slip and fall. Make sure the rest of your clothing is not too tight or heavy, as these cause over-heating.

Consider your workout area, especially if you are at home. Make sure you can move about, and not bump into any furniture. Your equipment also needs servicing regularly, as faulty machinery can be very dangerous. Your work out area must be clean, so as not to inhale nasty bacterial or viral infection.

Basic Human Physiology

Happy Healthy Hearts

Everyone knows that working out is good for the body. However, do you really understand the benefits between aerobics and heart health? Many people believe that doing aerobics if the best way for them to feel healthy and to be better in every aspect of their life. Aerobics and heart health is something to keep a check on; as it will help, you feel good and stay healthy.

The importance of aerobics and heart health is something that will undeniably stay with you for the rest of your life. The more aerobics you do the healthier your heart will become.

When it comes to the relationship between aerobics and your health, you give both your heart and lungs a workout. They work harder and faster. If you do aerobics daily, your heart and lungs will become stronger. Therefore, you will be able to do more aerobics without stopping.

You will have to work your way up. If you have not exercised for a while, your heart will not be strong enough to take too much. Take your time and talk to your doctor to develop and aerobics routine that will benefit you.

The Heart

An Introduction

The heart is an organ that pumps blood rich in oxygen to the body's cells. It is essential for human life. It beats approximately 80,000 to 100,000 per day, and pumps about 2000 gallons of blood to our muscles. The heart has to beat constantly to keep us alive.

The heart pumps blood into the arteries that carry oxygen to the body's cells. On the way back to the heart, the veins take deoxygenated blood to the lungs. Here the blood gathers oxygen again, and sends it back to the heart. This keeps the main blood circulation going.

The Heart's Structure

There are four chambers in the heart, consisting of two atria (singular; atrium) and two ventricles. It is pear-shaped and the size of a fist. It rests on the left side of the body, protected by the ribs. The heart's muscle or cardiac muscle categorized as an involuntary muscle, because we have no control over it.

The Three Layers of the Heart

PERICARDIUM
This layer contains a tough tissue that surrounds the heart. It splits into two layers:

Outer layer – this supports the heart and holds it in place by attaching to the chest cavity structures.

Inner layer – known also as the epicardium layer, is located on top of the heart muscle.

MYOCARDIUM

This layer is the cardiac muscle itself. It forms the walls of the four chambers.

ENDOCARDIUM

This layer comprises of thin endothelial and connective tissue. It looks white and shiny, and line the inner most layer. Its function is to prevent blood clots forming in the four chambers.

The Circulatory System

The superior vena cava brings de-oxygenated blood to the heart from the upper body, and the inferior vena cava brings it from the lower body. The vena cava is made of inelastic smooth muscle and feeds into the right atrium. Arteries are elastic, so they can withstand the pumping action.

Blood collects in the right atrium sent by the sinoatrial node in its upper wall. Both atria have to contract simultaneously to ensure the continuation of blood. The blood then passes through the tricuspid valve, allowing it to flow into the right ventricle. The valves allow the blood to pass, and stops any flowing back.

Now the blood is in the right ventricle via the AV node in the lower wall of the atrium. This node sends a signal via the Bundle of His to the Purkinje fibres, to

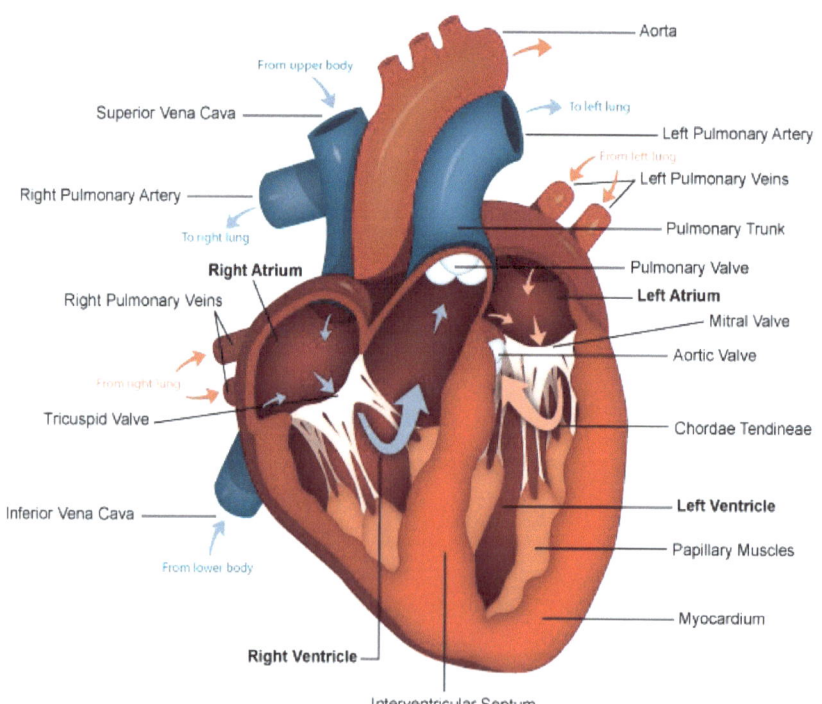

allow the ventricles to contract. The blood then flows out of the right ventricle through the pulmonary semilunar valve to the pulmonary artery, which takes it away from the heart. Again, the valves prevent the blood from flowing back into the ventricle.

The pulmonary artery is the only artery that carries de-oxygenated blood. It takes it out of the heart and the lungs. The extra blood causes the membrane surface of the lungs to increase due to their cellular sacs. These sacs named alveoli contain capillaries. The de-oxygenated blood now passes through these capillaries and re-oxygenated as we inhale oxygen. As we exhale, we release the carbon dioxide back into the air.

This process in the lungs is the so-called gaseous exchange. It converts carbon dioxide that come from the heart and body back into oxygen. The blood passes into the pulmonary vein, which takes this newly oxygenated blood back to the heart.

The oxygenated blood collects in the right atrium, causing the atrium walls to contract. It then passes through the mitral or bicuspid valve into the left ventricle.

The left ventricle then collects the blood that causes its walls to contract, allowing the blood to pass the aortic semilunar valve into the aorta.

The aorta is the largest artery to carry oxygenated blood away from the heart to the rest of the body. Not all the blood supplies the body, a little stays behind to supply the heart muscle with oxygen. This allows it to keep pumping.

When the body's cells are re-oxygenated and the blood has picked up the carbon dioxide, it will make it back to the heart via the vena cava.

How the Heart Beats

The two types of heartbeat are:

DIASTOLE – During this type of heartbeat, the thick muscular walls of the ventricles relax, causing pressure to drop. The bicuspid valve opens allowing the atria to full up with blood. Then the valve contacts, allowing blood to flow into the ventricles, causing them to expand. The blood pressure in the aorta decreases, and the semi-lunar valve closes.

SYSTOLE – During this type of heartbeat, the thick muscular walls of the ventricles start to contract, causing pressure to rise. The bicuspid and tricuspid valves close. Blood pumps through the aorta to the pulmonary artery, and the atria relax. The left atrium receives blood via the pulmonary vein, and the right atrium from the vena cava.

<u>Heart Rate</u>

It is important to know your heart rate when exercising. It will help you to notice if you are doing the right exercises, and doing them correctly. If you are new to exercise, your ideal heart rate will be in the region of 50-60% of your maximum heart rate. Remember to use warm up exercises before starting your routine. Building up your rate gradually will help reduce body fat, lower blood pressure and cholesterol levels and therefore burn 85% of your body's calories. If you are a fit person and used to exercise, your target heart rate is about 60-70% of your maximum heart rate. This will ensure quicker weight loss and that you burn more calories. The ideal heart rate is around 70-80%.

TABLE TO SHOW TARGET HEART RATES IN BEATS PER MINUTE

AGE	TARGET RANGE (BEATS/MINUTE)
20-24	120-150
25-29	117-146
30-34	114-142
35-39	111-139
40-44	108-135
45-49	105-131
50-54	102-127
55-59	99-123
60-64	96-120
65-69	93-116
70+	90-113

Aerobics Trims the Heart

After years of research on the effects on the heart, they eventually produced some amazing results. By regularly, doing aerobics you can reduce an enlarged heart. A trimmer heart means that it is a more effective organ for pumping blood. A further study was performed on patients suffering from heart failure. The results showed that if the patient worked out several times a week, their hearts began to pump better.

In the USA alone there are about five million people suffering from heart failure. This leads to large numbers of people being hospitalized causing costs to the health service in the region of thirty billion dollars.

If someone suffers from years of heart failure, these people usually suffer from high blood pressure that can eventually lead to a heart attack. You develop an enlarged heart, which is out of shape and eventually becomes too weak to pump.

For many years, doctors would avoid prescribing exercise to patients with heart failure. They used to give plenty of best rest to relieve the extra stress on the heart instead. During the last decade, research has found that exercise is good. It reduces the symptoms of heart failure, and reverses the effects of harmful hormones. These improvements help to compensate some of the weakness formed in the heart.

The extra oxygen that enters the heart during aerobics causes chemical transformation. The heart can now pump oxygenated blood through the body more effectively. The body's lung capacity increases, allowing more oxygen to enter the body. Oxygen strengthens the heart muscle, so that the body can detoxify better, reducing the risk of illness. This activity of the heart increases HDL that removes the bad cholesterol from the blood.

Aerobics can lower the blood pressure so the heart maximizes our work, but we do it with effort, enabling the body to feel fit, avoid illness, have no lethargy and enjoy a better, clearer memory.

Heart and Lungs Work Together

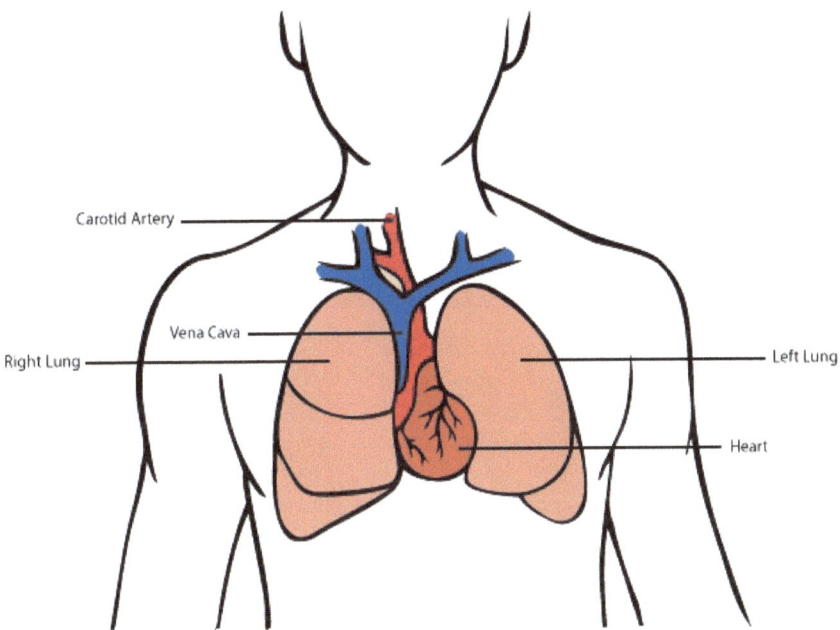

When you are doing exercise, more blood will be flowing into your muscles. It will increase about four to five times that of resting rate.

The sympathetic nerve stimulates the respiratory muscles to increase their breathing rate. The metabolic by-products (waste), such as lactic acid, hydrogen ions and carbon dioxide stimulate the brainstem's nerve centres to activate the muscles. Blood pressure then rises with increased heartbeat and cardiac output opening the outlets to the alveoli in the lungs. This will of course, increase ventilation bringing more oxygen into the blood, to help muscles work to their full capacity.

When resting 5 litres of blood flow every minute.

(0.07L x 70 Beat per minute = 4.9 L per minute).

As blood flow increases, it pumps 20-25 litres per minute.

The Lungs
The Structure of the Lungs

Diagram of the Human Lungs

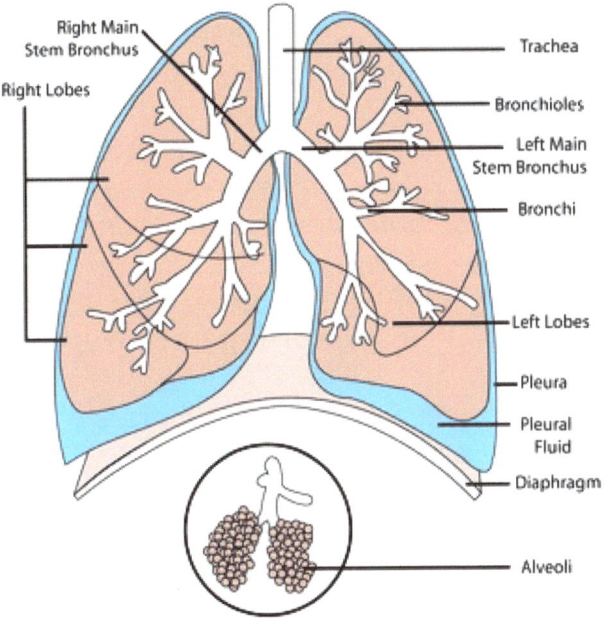

The trachea or windpipe is made up of mostly cartilage, which helps to keep the trachea permanently open. The trachea passes down the thorax and connects the larynx (contains the vocal cords) with the bronchi, which pass into the lungs.

The bronchi (singular; bronchus) are two short tubes, similar in structure to the trachea, which carry air into each lung. They are lined with a mucous membrane and ciliated cells and, like the trachea, contain cartilage to hold them open. The mucous traps solid particles and cilia (tiny hair like structures) and moves it upwards, preventing dirt entering the delicate lung tissue. The bronchi subdivide into bronchioles in the lungs. These subdivide, yet again, and finally end in minute air-filled sacs called alveoli (singular; alveolus).

The lungs are cone-shaped, spongy organs situated in the thoracic cavity on either side of the heart. Internally, the lungs consist of tiny air sacs called alveoli, which are arranged in lobules and resemble "grapes". The function of the lungs is to facilitate the exchange of the gases, oxygen and carbon dioxide, and in order to carry this out efficiently the lungs have several important features:

- A very large surface area provided by the alveoli.
- A thin permeable membrane surrounding the walls of the alveoli.
- A thin film of water lining the alveoli, which is essential for dissolving the oxygen from the alveoli air.
- Thin walled blood capillaries forming a network around the alveoli, which absorb oxygen from the air breathed into the lungs and release carbon dioxide into the air breathed out of the alveoli.

The Mechanics of Respiration

Inspiration/Inhaling

1. Intercostal muscles found between the ribs contract and pull the ribs up and out.
2. The diaphragm muscle contracts, moving down and outwards.
3. Due to steps 1 and 2 above, the size of the thoracic cavity increases, because of the reduced pressure within. Air rushes in and the lungs become inflated.

Expiration/Exhaling

1. The intercostal muscles relax and the ribs fall and go in.
2. The diaphragm relaxes and becomes dome shaped.
3. Due to steps, 1 and 2 above, the thoracic cavity is now smaller and because of the increased pressure up it air rushes out and the lungs become deflated.

How Haemoglobin Works

Haemoglobin is a protein that binds to red blood cells as they carry most of the oxygen and carbon dioxide around the body. It first binds to carbon dioxide as the haemoglobin enters the lungs. Oxygen levels become high, as carbon dioxide levels decrease.

Haemoglobin then binds to the new oxygen. It is then transported through the heart on its way to the body's muscles. Here the body's metabolism causes carbon dioxide levels to rise, as oxygen decreases due to it being released as energy. Again, the carbon dioxide binds to the carbon dioxide transporting back to the lungs where the whole process is recycled.

During exercise, the metabolic activity of the body is high due to the muscles working harder. This increases the waste products of hydrogen ions and lactic acid. It causes the local pH (balance of acid and alkaline) levels to be lower than normal. Therefore, the attraction of oxygen and haemoglobin is reduced, as more oxygen has to be released in the muscle to enable it to work harder.

Asthma and Exercise

Sufferers of asthma usually think that they cannot exercise properly or safely, because of their condition. Asthmatics can get in shape and exercise. Many well-known athletes and sports personalities suffer from asthma, and are still able to compete. So do not be discouraged, take your encouragement from them. (Names cannot be mentioned here, but you can research this on the internet if you need more information).

Asthma is a chronic lung disease that shows symptoms of coughing, wheezing, shortness of breath and chest tightness. It tends to occur in people where it is hereditary or who are allergic to environmental pollutants. Well-known triggers are exposure to allergens, such as pollen, dust mites and cockroaches, viral respiratory infections, airway irritants and exercise.

How to Prevent Attacks

1. Try to bathe your pets weekly.
2. Do not smoke or allow smoking in your home.
3. If possible, when mould and pollen counts are high, stay indoors and use the air medication available these days to help with airborne allergies. Take advantage of these, if you can, and give yourself a normal life. See your doctor about it today.
4. Wash bedding and stuffed toys regularly in hot water.
5. Wash your hands often, so that allergens from your hands do not get near your face, which will set off symptoms.
6. Get a flu jab.
7. Wear a scarf over your mouth and nose during winter months.

8.	Get to know your triggers and how to avoid them.

Now that you know what asthma is, you may be wondering how exercise fits in. Most doctors will not tell you to give up exercise or sport. You just have to take special precautions to avoid attacks. Keep your inhaler and medication close. Never use your inhaler more than three times during physical activity. If your symptoms persist, stop what you are doing, and maybe contact your doctor if the symptoms do not go away.

If your asthma keeps you awake during the night with coughing and wheezing, only do light exercise the next day.

For *Exercise Induced Asthma (EIA)*, symptoms usually appear about 6 – 10 minutes of starting exercise. They get worse during cold or dry air. If you suffer from this type of asthma, you can still enjoy swimming, walking, biking, downhill skiing and team based sports.

Remember, asthma is "not in your head"; it is a real medical condition that requires preventative treatment. Take your medication everywhere, and be proactive.

DO NOT HAVE A MISERABLE LIFE WITH ASTHMA; ENJOY EXERCISE JUST LIKE EVERY ONE ELSE!

Eliminating Waste Products

Even though it is good for our bodies, exercise uses a lot of energy and produces many waste products. For example, it increases the amount of lactic acid in our bodies. Lactic acid forms when the muscles do not receive enough oxygen, and they begin to break down glucose. While it may help muscles to contract more efficiently, it can sometimes make muscles sore for days after exercising. In addition to lactic acid, our bodies will have an excess amount of carbon dioxide, adenosine and hydrogen ions. All of these things can be beneficial in small quantities, but are considered waste products when they reach a certain level. Once they cross the threshold into excess amounts, the bloodstream is responsible for getting rid of them.

Producing Body Heat

When exercise is taking place, the body takes the elements that are already present within and break them down. Lactic acid forms from the breakdown of the sugars within the body. This releases a fair amount of energy, but it is only chemical energy. The body will then take the energy formed from the chemical reactions taking place inside of it and transform it into a type of mechanical energy. This mechanical energy is what makes the muscles contract more efficiently. It could even result in better endurance because the muscles and tissues will have so much more mechanical energy. Over time, this mechanical energy will convert into heat energy, which explains why we become overheated as exercise progresses.

The heat energy causes the blood vessels to dilate. As the passageways within the vessels open up, they allow an increased amount of blood to flow through them. The increased amount of blood causes the skin to feel hotter. The body cannot function properly with that level of heat inside of it, so it must find some way to cool itself. Sweat cools the body down by releasing the heat through fluids.

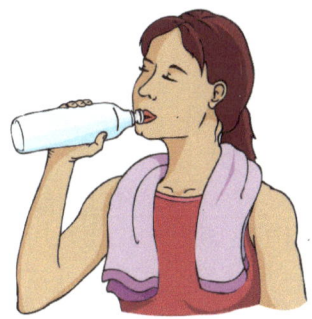

However, sweat does not happen automatically. The brain cannot physically communicate with every part of the body, because of its location in the head. Instead, it communicates with different receptor sites within the body. These will in turn send various messages to the brain to let it know that they body is not functioning properly. In this case, it will tell the brain that it needs to find some way to release all of the built-up heat energy. The part of the brain responsible for the body's thermostat is known as the hypothalamus. The hypothalamus can stimulate the body to generate more heat or it can send the proper signals to release heat.

The hypothalamus signals the sweat glands to begin collecting heat energy and releasing it through fluids. The sweat that comes of the body carries the heat with it and helps to cool the body down. However, this will lead to a decrease in fluids present in the body. It is very important to continue drinking plenty of fluids during exercise or the body could become dehydrated. Water is a great choice for this, but sports drinks can also have a great effect on the body. Sports drinks tend to supply additional ingredients that restore the body to its proper levels, such as sodium and potassium ions, as well as more glucose or sugars.

Heat Stroke

Sometimes the body has a difficult time cooling itself down and can seriously overheat. This is a type of hyperthermia known as a heat stroke. Those who work outdoors, who participate in athletics, infants or the elderly tend to be at a greater risk for developing a heat stroke. A heat stroke alters the way the nervous system functions, making it incredibly dangerous. It is very different from a less severe form of hyperthermia known as heat exhaustion. The symptoms of heat exhaustion include nausea, vomiting, dizziness, weakness, headaches, fatigue or muscle cramps.

When it comes to a heat stroke, the symptoms become much more severe. They may include high body temperature, confusion, hallucinations, agitated behaviours or disorientation. Another common symptom is the absence of sweating, even though the skin is hot and flushed. A rapid pulse or difficulties of breathing are some of the first indicators of a heat stroke. If not treated quickly, they could result in seizures or comas. The symptoms that are experienced can vary from person to person. While these are the most common, not everyone who is having a heat stroke will exhibit all of these symptoms.

It is important to take immediate action when a heat stroke develops. The most important thing to do for a heat stroke victim is to attempt to cool them down. This could involve placing ice packs on their body, particularly under their arms or over their groin. You could fan them to help ward off the body heat. If they are able, you may attempt to have them drink some cool water or sports drink. If available, you may even spray them with a hose to help release their body heat.

Monitor their body temperature until it drops to 38.3 to 38.8 C.

It is always important to contact emergency services when this occurs. Continue the cooling process until an ambulance arrives. They may even provide you with additional instructions upon calling them. Heat stroke is a severe problem and should be treated as such. Many who go untreated end in fatalities.

Body Fat

Everybody needs a certain amount of fat in order for the body to function properly. The body develops this fat through fatty acids and adipose tissues. Fat cells are unique because they can form a variety of different things. They can produce fat tissue, fatty acids and adipose. Fatty acids form when long chains of fats are broken down inside the body. These fatty acids are healthy because the body can use them as an energy source. Adipose tissue is tissue where fat is stored, typically in the form of triglycerides. This adipose tissue can take two forms, depending on the place in the body and the age of the person.

White adipose tissue is responsible for three primary functions. It insulates the body, providing a certain amount of heat. When the body does not have enough energy intake to equal the amount of energy that it is using, white adipose can convert into a source of energy. The body can break it down and use it to create a mechanical energy. Furthermore, it also provides a certain amount of mechanical cushioning. It surrounds certain organs and provides a means of protection for them. This type of tissue is more commonly found in adults.

The other type of adipose tissue is known as brown tissue. This is the most common type of fat found in new-borns. The other place where brown tissue collects is between their shoulder blades. While the white tissue is responsible for insulating the body, brown tissue is responsible for thermogenesis. This means that the brown tissue is part of the reason that our bodies maintain a stable temperature. This tissue is what keeps us from shivering on a regular basis while our bodies find warmth.

Fat Entering the Body

Fat enters the body through the things that we eat. Whenever fatty foods are consumed, the body stores the bits that it does not use immediately as triglycerides. Triglycerides are a type of lipid found in fat cells that can have some detrimental health side effects. Too many triglycerides could cause unwanted heart problems later on in life. The stomach and the small intestine cannot digest triglycerides, and they get stored as fatty tissue throughout the body.

When fatty foods are consumed, the body attempts a process known as emulsification. Emulsification is the process where the body attempts to break down the fat that has entered the body. Large areas of fat mix with bile salts directly from the gall bladder. This will cause them to break down into smaller drops, known as micelle drops. As this happens, the surface area of the fats increases, which allows for a greater chance at digestion. Lipases, or enzymes that secrete from the pancreas, will attack the newly formed micelles. This will cause them to break down into both glycerol (which can be a type of triglyceride) and fatty acids. They will be absorbed into the intestine lining.

Triglycerides now begin to form, covered in a protein coating. The fat molecules that the body could not immediately use are being stored elsewhere in the body. The new lipids that are formed, namely chylomicrons, are a special type of protein. They dissolve far more easily in water, which is one of the primary elements in the bloodstream. It is more likely to enter the bloodstream for use in this way. However, the chylomicrons do not survive for a long period of time. The lipoprotein lipase, which supports enzyme breakdown, will again transform it into a fatty acid.

The fatty acids have very few places to go once they are formed in the body. For the most part, much of it is stored in the blood vessels and heart muscle. The fatty acids will line the walls of the blood vessels, making it difficult for blood to pump through. Other times, they will get stored up in the heart muscle as storage. Neither option promotes good cardiovascular health. They will later be released into the lymphatic system. They are too big for the tiny capillary walls, where veins and arteries merge. Instead, they will pass into the blood as a type of drainage system.

Fat Storage

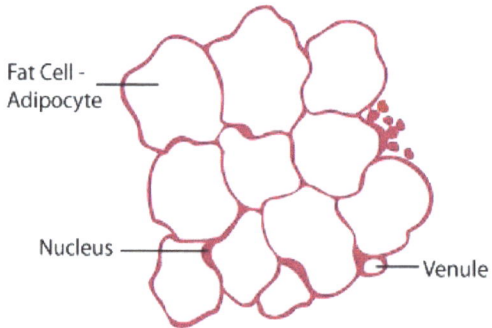

The amounts of fat cells that a person has will never multiply or grow larger, even as they seem to gain weight. Instead, the cell itself will begin to carry more and more of the droplets of fat that were formed during the digestive process.   Instead of increasing in number, the fat cells increase in size and take up a greater amount of space within the body.   When a person starts to lose weight, some of the fat droplets that are in these cells will disappear, but they will always have the same amount of cells.   The average person could have anywhere from 50 to 200 billion of these fat cells. Majority of them lay directly under the skin, but they may accumulate in various areas.

For females, it is more common for fat cells to become distributed around the breasts, hips, waist and buttocks areas. Males tend to accumulate them in the abdomen, chest and buttocks regions. However, these are the only places where we can visibly see the storage of fat. Many times, they also surround internal organs, such as the liver, kidneys, and inside muscle. The fat that surrounds organs acts as a cushion so that they are not jarred during physical activity. The fat that is stored inside muscle gives the muscle more volume, but without proper exercise, the amount of fat within the muscle could surpass the amount of muscle and lead to a decrease in strength.

Insulin

The body has a difficult time processing glucose on its own, so it uses a special chemical known as insulin. Whenever you eat a meal, the body breaks it down into separate components, such as glucose, amino acids and fatty acids. Once these things reach the intestine where they must either be absorbed for use by the body or excreted, the intestine will stimulate the production and release of the hormone insulin. Insulin is stored in the pancreas and released to help the body to use these various parts of food.

It will absorb the glucose, amino acids and fatty acids. However, it will then stop breaking down these elements and they will become an entirely new component. For example, the glucose will be turned into fats, the fatty acids and glycerol will become a type of protein, and the amino acids will be left alone for the body to use. It will help to build glycogen from the glucose, fats (or triglycerides) from the glycerol, fatty acids and proteins from the amino acids. Glycogen is a form of carbohydrate stored in the body for later use or energy expenditure. The fatty acids that were originally present become stored in the blood fat cells, the muscle cells or the liver cells. The insulin helps to break down the fat molecules and store them as fat drops within cells.

Fat Breakdown

The body is constantly using energy, which comes mainly from its internal stores of carbohydrates, fats and proteins. When you are not eating, it means that you are not absorbing food or energy. There will be a low insulin level in the blood, which helps to break down the fatty acids and convert them into useable energy. Organs within the body, particularly those within the endocrine system, begin to secrete hormones, which work in the opposite way of insulin. For example, the pancreas will secrete glucagon. The pituitary gland will release the growth hormone ACTH, or the adrenocorticotropic hormone. The adrenal gland releases epinephrine, better known as adrenaline. The thyroid gland will secrete thyroid hormones, the most common of which are triiodothyronine and thyroxine.

All of these hormones work together on the liver, muscle, fat and tissue within the body. The body's primary source of energy is always glucose. However, if the body is not eating, it must begin to break down some of the fats that are stored away into glucose. In a process known as glycogenolysis, the carbohydrates and the glycogen that are stored away in the body will begin to form simple sugars in order to give energy to the rest of the cells. Next, the body will break down the fats into glycerol and fatty acids. This is called lipolysis. When the internal stores are broken down this way, it leads to an increase in energy. However, if the body does not need energy immediately and it needs glucose instead, lipolysis could be one of the first steps of gluconeogenesis, the process of creating glucose from fatty acids and amino acids.

Losing Weight and Fat

Weight can be broken down into a simple formula that explains how we either gain or lose weight. It is the rate at which we consume food, and store energy, compared to the amount of energy that we use. When we use more energy than we have stored, we lose weight. The opposite is also true: when we store more energy than we use, then we will gain weight. The number of fat cells will always be the same, but they can increase and decrease in size. There are generally considered to be three rules for losing weight and fat.

The first important thing to remember when trying to maintain your weight is to eat a balanced diet. This includes carbohydrates, proteins, and fats because all of these things are good for the body. They help to store up energy in case you may need it at a later time. The second important thing is to make sure that you are not overeating. Having an excess of energy stored away will lead to an increase in weight and fat. Anywhere from 1,500 to 2,000 calories a day is normally sufficient for a relatively active person. The last rule to maintaining a proper weight is to exercise regularly. This helps to prevent the build-up of stored fats and it keeps muscles toned and healthy.

Targeting the Abdomen

When attempting to work out or lose weight, sometimes it is best to target one particular area of the body at a time. The abdomen is a great place to start, as it helps with many of our central movements. The abdomen is the set of muscles from the chest to the pelvis, most of which helps us to stretch and move around. The muscles here can protect organs such as the stomach and intestine from receiving a significant amount of damage. They also help with regular body functions, such as defecation or urination. It is important to work out these muscles so that the body can stay healthy.

One of the most important things to think about and remember during exercise is to repeat the motions. Repetition helps to build up muscle endurance and builds up muscle faster. It is also important to add stretches to the routine. Stretches keep the muscles from becoming too sore and inflexible. When the muscles move more regularly, the movement of the body becomes so much easier. It can also improve posture and decrease tension that can quickly accumulate during a hard workout.

When it comes time for the actual exercise, all movements should come directly from the abdomen. This keeps unnecessary pressure off your back, shoulders, knees, neck or any other joint that may experience discomfort otherwise. The most common type of abdominal exercise is the crunch. To perform a crunch, you lie on the floor with your knees bent and feet placed firmly on the ground. With the hands behind your head, you use your abdominal muscles to pull yourself up towards your knees. The pressure should not be on your neck or back, but should stem from your abdomen. The same thing can also be done with variations. For example, you could keep your arms straight out in a continuous line of your upper body. You could also raise your feet up to form a ninety-degree angle.

Another good abdomen workout is a plank. You get into a push-up position, with arms located directly under the shoulders and the rest of your body in a straight line. The abdomen muscles should help you to stay in this position. This can also be modified by resting your elbows on the ground underneath your shoulders. This exercise can be held for brief periods of time and then repeated in order to strengthen muscles.

Diet and Exercise

A proper diet is necessary for growth and weight maintenance. It is important to consume the right foods so that the muscles will have the correct energy and fuel that they need to continue to sustain daily functioning. The most important things that muscles need in order to function properly are glucose and glycogen. The body can convert several different things into both glucose and glycogen, which it will later store for future use. Good examples of foods that are rich in these two elements are bread, pasta, rice, and several different cuts of meat. Ripe fruits and vegetables will also have a high amount of glucose that occurs naturally, but processed foods and juices may have glucose included as well.

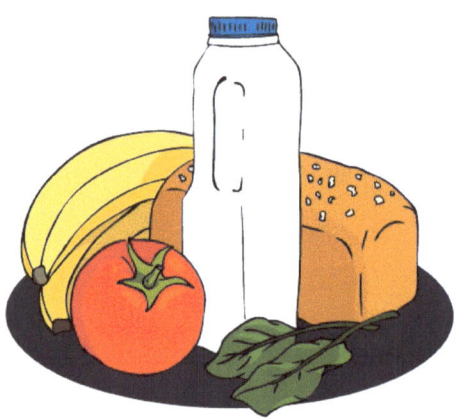

The liver plays a crucial role in the storage and maintenance of glycogen. It can hold up to ten percent of its volume in glycogen, so this is where a lot of it becomes stored. Here, the liver will monitor the amount of sugar present in the bloodstream. When it deems it necessary, it will release some of its stored glycogen into the body. Glycogen can also be stored in the muscles. The muscles will hold on to it until they need to use more energy than they currently have. The glycogen can be broken down into pieces that allow it to generate more energy.

Weight range is typically measured by the ratio of weight to height. This ratio is known as the body mass index or BMI. When BMI is anywhere from 25 to 29.9, a person is considered overweight. At a BMI of 30 or more, they will be considered obese. A normal weight range is between the 18.5 and 24.9 BMI. Anything lower than 18.5 is considered to be underweight.

In general, fat or adipose tissue is found directly beneath the skin. This is called subcutaneous fat. While this is the most common placement and storage of fat, it also tends to gather in other places. For example, much of it will gather on top of the kidneys, within muscles and in the liver. The hormones in the body make the fat distribution different in males and females. For example, men will have more fat in their chest, abdomen and buttocks. Women will accumulate more fat in their breasts, hips, waist and buttocks.

Crunches are a great way to get rid of excess fat and strengthen the abdominal muscles. To perform a crunch, rest with your back on the floor, knees bent, and feet placed firmly on the ground. With the hands underneath the head and arms out to the sides, use your abdominal muscles to draw yourself upwards. Using the same muscles, slowly lower yourself back to the ground. This can be repeated until you feel as though your abdomen has had a good workout.

Push-ups are great for both abdominal strength and upper body strength. Lie on the floor with hands directly under the shoulders and push yourself up. Your toes should be on the floor and hands flat, while the rest of your body is being supported. Slowly lower yourself until your chest touches the ground and push yourself back up again. This can also be repeated for the best effects.

Lunges are another great exercise for helping to build the muscles in your legs. Stand with feet placed together. Take one-step forward and lower your body down until your front leg is bent at a ninety-degree angle. Come back up and place both feet back together again. Make sure to repeat this on both sides of your body.

While these are some simple exercises that can help to burn unwanted fat and tone muscles, you can do several other things as well. For example, taking a brisk walk or jog is sure to burn some calories and help your body get into shape. This raises your heart rate and burns energy, which reduces the amount of stored fat within fat cells.

Benefits of Exercise

Besides helping to keep your body looking healthy, exercise has some great long-term health benefits associated with it. For many people, exercise and regular workouts can be a great stress-reliever. It helps them to channel frustrations and stresses from throughout the day and turns them into something positive. Because of this, it can help people to tolerate anxiety, stress and depression in a healthier way. People who report regular exercise routines generally have a more positive outlook on life.

Apart from the mental side effects of exercise, there are many health reasons to consider as well. For example, exercising reduces high blood pressure. The heart learns to work more efficiently when it is exercised with aerobics on a regular basis. Not to mention, there is a large reduction in weight loss seen with regular exercise. This means that the fat cells within in the body are growing smaller. It also means that there is not as much fat build-up around the heart and inside the blood vessels. This helps with health overall. Exercise can also control cholesterol. It controls the lipid level in the body and helps to reduce it until it is at a healthy level. It also prevents and control diabetes, as well as reducing the risk for colon cancer.

However, sometimes exercise encourages people to make healthier choices. Many people find that they are more committed to quitting smoking once they start an exercise routine. It will also improve muscle flexibility, making daily movements much easier. Bones and joints are more flexible, which could lead to greater comfort with movement later in life.

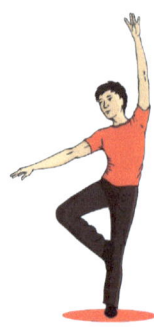

Exercise could be as simple as going for a walk in the evenings or it could require a bit more time. A good option for a regular workout is to join a sports team, such as soccer, football, basketball, tennis or cross-country.

However, there are also individual sports like horseback riding, dance, ice-skating and gymnastics. Some sports can be both a great hobby and a beneficial workout for your body. It could be a healthy way to spend your free time, and something that you enjoy. If joining a team seems too expensive, perhaps joining a simple class on occasion would be a good option. Some classes are offered regularly, such as yoga, Pilates and aerobics. Joining a class could be a great way to make new friends and become healthier.

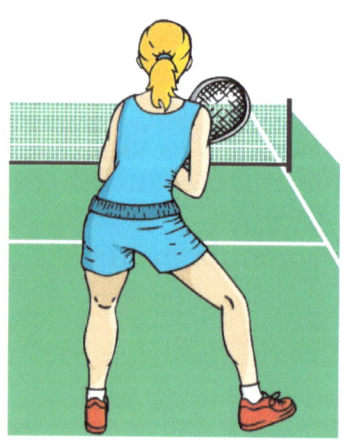

Consulting a Doctor

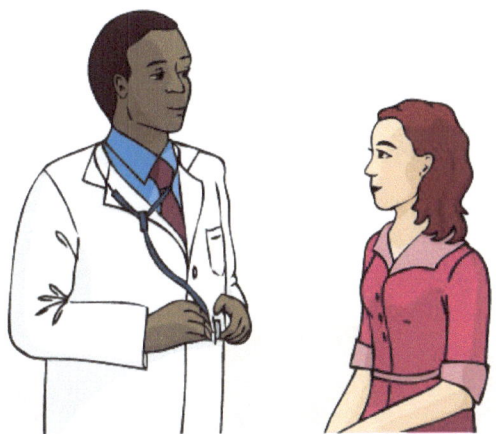

Sometimes it is necessary to consult a doctor before beginning a new exercise program. There are so many beneficial side effects to exercise that it may seem harmless to begin immediately. However, some people have pre-existing conditions that could result in a range of dangerous side effects if they not exercise properly or put too much stress on the body. They may need to consult a doctor to determine if a particular type of exercise is well suited to their condition.

Some of these conditions include heart disease, asthma, lung disease, diabetes, liver disease, kidney disease or arthritis. People who experience these problems need to be especially careful with their medical health when considering their exercise regimen. If you believe that you may have any type of heart or lung problem, you may also decide to consult a doctor first. Some of these symptoms include a heart murmur, swelling in the ankles, dizziness, shortness of breath even when resting, pain in the chest, jaw, neck or arms when exercising, or muscle pain that subsides once exercise is over.

Trainers sometimes recommend consulting a doctor prior to beginning something new depending on lifestyle instead of diseases or other medical conditions. For example, many say that if you smoke, have not worked out in three months or more or are over the age of 45 for men or 55 for women, it would be in your best interest to make sure it is medically safe for you to proceed. If you are overweight, obese, have pre-diabetes, high blood pressure or high cholesterol, a doctor may also be of great help in determining what type of exercise would be most beneficial for your lifestyle.

Some pain and muscle soreness is to be expected from exercise. Sometimes, the pain felt during exercise is a good indicator that you should consult a doctor before continuing your exercises. Any type of pain or pressure on the left side of your head, neck, chest or arms is not a good sign. If you feel dizzy, sick, or break out into a cold sweat, it may seem like nothing, but it could be a sign that there is a larger problem. Furthermore, any muscle cramps, sharp pains in your feet, joints, or bones, or irregular or rapid heartbeats should warrant some type of medical supervision or consultation.

Many injuries that require medical attention should be noted through the amount of pain that you perceive. For example, a sprained ankle or wrist will be very painful. If you experience something that gives you a great deal of pain, it is probably best to err on the side of caution and seek a medical opinion.

Other Books by Cindy Wright

Travelling Through the Emerald Isle

A Journey through the Histories of the Provinces of the
Republic of Ireland
By Cindy Wright

Take a journey back in time with Travelling through the Emerald Isle. Learn about the histories of the cities that are prominent attractions in Ireland. This book details the histories of various areas and places located through the provinces of Leinster, Connaught, Munster and Ulster, including Galway, Dublin and Roscommon. The stories are perfect for anyone who is thinking of travelling to Ireland or someone who just thirsts for the knowledge of the land.

Worlds of Ice - A Guide to the Life and History of the Arctic and Antarctic

By Cindy Wright

This brief textbook gives in-depth detail of the types of life forms that are commonly discovered in the Arctic Circle and around the continent of Antarctica. It provides rich information about specific animals, both those living on the land and in the icy waters. It is perfect for anyone wishing to expand their knowledge of the fauna in these ecosystems. Written with enough detail to inform those who are new to Arctic studies of the minor subtleties of life in this area, it is a great starting point for those thirsting to know of these worlds. It is a great book, whether you have previous knowledge or not!

Part of Your World - Practical Earth Science Knowledge for the Real World

By Cindy Wright

This brief textbook offers an easy to understand, comprehensive overview of the most important topics related to earth science today. From astronomy to geology, it covers everything you might need to know for real world application. It features up-to-date information on important topics that everyone should understand. Its primary goal is to help students to increase their knowledge, but it is also perfect for those who have no experience in this area. It is a great place to start learning about how nature works!

Christmas Magic for Children

By Cindy Wright

Want to spread a little Christmas magic and joy with your children this Christmas, then this is the book for you. Written so that children will understand and enjoy from a very small age, even if read to. It introduces the history of certain Christmas traditions as well as old and popular songs. Included are short stories that will make it fun for the children and bring the magic alive. Not forgetting the pictures that the children can look at if being read to. Whether you want to learn about the first Christmas, when Jesus was born, or when Santa was first recognized for the gift bringer that he is known for today. You will also learn about Rudolph and his story, as well as Frosty our faithful snowman that comes back year after year when it snows. In this book, you will also get a summary of other historical traditions; such as when Christmas cards were first sent, and who were the first people to put up a Christmas tree in their home. To found out much, much more you will need to purchase the book.

SPREAD THE MAGIC, WHICH IS AVAILABLE FOR CHILDREN FROM 1 -100+.

The Different Ways of Celebrating Easter

By Cindy Wright

Christmas may have come and gone for another year, but next up is Easter. Whether you are a Christian celebrating the crucifixion of Jesus or looking forward to all those Easter eggs. Maybe both!

Here is a book to get you in the mood. Filled with facts, stories and poems. Suitable for all ages, whether you are a child or a grown up. Learn about the tradition of Easter and celebrate in style.

www.ingramcontent.com/pod-product-compliance
Lightning Source LLC
Chambersburg PA
CBHW050821290526
45792CB00001B/210